Me & My Tourette's

Me & My Tourette's

✦

Motivated by GOD

Written, Typed, & Biography By
Myles R. Walker

iUniverse, Inc.
New York Lincoln Shanghai

Me & My Tourette's
Motivated by GOD

iUniverse books may be ordered through booksellers or by contacting:

iUniverse
2021 Pine Lake Road, Suite 100
Lincoln, NE 68512
www.iuniverse.com
1-800-Authors (1-800-288-4677)

ISBN-13: 978-0-595-39058-8 (pbk)
ISBN-13: 978-0-595-83446-4 (ebk)
ISBN-10: 0-595-39058-7 (pbk)
ISBN-10: 0-595-83446-9 (ebk)

Printed in the United States of America

Contents

The Author

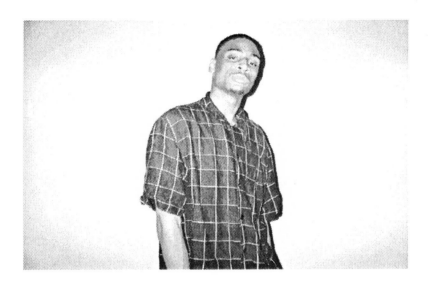

Hi yall doin out there in readers world. Hi my name is Myles R. Walker I'm a 24 year old African American Male who's been living with Tourette Syndrome for 17yrs. I really don't want to do this biography about myself because I don't want this biography to look like I'm applying for a J-O-B or sound like a cheesy way to scoop a hot date. Biographies are like short story intro's that tell a lil bit about that person(s) who wrote the book, and in this case it's me who's thee culprit.

This book was is the very first book to be written a year and a half ago, and it most certainly won't be the last of many to come. It has just been published this year in April 2006. I love God. He's always been there throughout my life.

I Love to Drive, so put me behind the wheel of any automobile and watch me peel out. Driving is a passion that I've had since I was little, which came from my Grandmother 1LUV. Why? Because we both have medical condi-

tions Big Up Grand Ma. I adore the great outdoors. I'm a musician who plays the drums, I constantly write poetry, rhymes, songs, and enjoy taking pictures. Just call me a "Black Renaissance Man"

I love children, cooking, dogs. Some of my many hobbies are watching television, sports I consider myself as an All American meaning "I love em all A to Z and I would actively involve myself in them on or off the field. When It comes to movies, I should be the Black Ebert/Ropert thumbs way up, I study pretty decently when it come to movies cuz that is what I want to do among other things.

Traveling is a must I can't stay put I need to explore and see the sights from the Projects to the Penthouse, 20,000 leagues under the sea to space let's go somewhere. I'm very comfortable in my own skin, and know how to have fun out in public and/or in privacy on my own surroundings.

Spending time with my immediate family which is my Mother, Brother, Grandparents and Uncle is of great substance no matter what. "Heeeey yooou Guuys!

I hoped that you have enjoyed this Bio intro about me you'll learn more soon or later. Love and live Live Life to the Fullest Everyday is a Holiday!!

I want too Thank God for God, and for being their every step of the way. In the beginning, when no one else has, or ever will be. Also for the gift of a medical condition called Tourette Syndrome, for which I love and cherish sincerely.

For never deserting us 3, for taking care of me and my 2 favorite family members in the whole wide world, in and out of Heaven, Hell, Space and the Universe, that my life has been living around 20+ years thus far.

I Thank God for my Mother "Warrior Gloria" for her God given fighting spirit, her realness, for being such an Ancient Being, for nurturing, bearing, feeding, carrying and laboring 9 months of reproduction 2 babies. Loving, fighting, helping, and pushing my brother and me and all others in life that needs a Warrior like her.

My brother Robert AKA "Frogge or Skillet Head", for loving me and my Tourette Syndrome and not making me feel low down because of my disability when all others have rejected and disrespected me. For becoming an Intellectual individual who corrects me when I am wrong and need it, as well as turning me into your little brother and becoming my Big Brother B-4 day 1 You were meant for me and I was meant for you Dude!! Holla Back Young 'N'

God Bless You 2 for loving me the way I was built, sticking with me through thick-N-thin, never ever turning your backs against the wall on me like a whole lot of shady people, You 2 Guys are the match made from Heaven that God conjured up and knew that us 3 would fit very well Together. After God and His Son Jesus! "You 2 are The 3rd most needed substance in my Life to keep me smiling and walking on my toes and you cannot Ever!, Ever!, Ever!, Ever!, Ever!, Ever!, Ever! Be Replaced. No matter what I, do, say, try, accomplish, achieve, seek out, good or bad, from top to bottom, bottom to top, U-2 are some TRU Ruff Ryders.

The words that I say and speak mean absolutely nothing; expression doesn't know what each one of you is about!! "Aright I aint gone talk"

Introduction

This is my first book that I have ever written and produced for myself in life. "I don't care what none of you's think I just do me". If you Like it~~ Holla Back, if not Let me see you do a better job! Now!!......

Time to get comfy people,

So make something to drink that will soothe your taste buds. Grab your slippers, your reading glasses; get your night robe, pajamas or any other pair of clothing that puts you at ease when you read. Dim the lights, jusss Blaze some candles, pull the shades down, get the batteries and load up the flashlights.

I'm just trying to put you readers in that readers mode. Am I doing too much?? No? Well then, find a comfortable spot, get cozy, sit back relax and

~ENJOY~

1

I want to shed some light from myself, about being a 20+ years old African-American Man who has lived with Tourette Syndrome since the tender age of 7. I want you to see, feel, imagine, and experience the up's, downs, ins and outs that I've been through with this condition. Anywhere from being accepted by few to rejected by many.

I Thank God that I have this type of condition, and I love my Tourette's, I really do! I am truly glad that we are still together after all of these years and can never ever be torn apart, unless the Good Lord in Heaven above wants me to be healed! I love my Tourette's so much more now than I ever did before in my childhood days. If I do say so myself, I honestly believe that this is one of the best thing's that has ever happened to me!

Inhale, exhale, inhale, exhale, breathe slowly yall! Anybody out there in need of some CPR?? You people alright out there?? Just checking, just trying to see if you are still with me. I know a lot of you are in a state of shock or disbelief after hearing such a bold statement that may seem unorthodox or obnoxious to those of you that do not understand the sincerity of my true feelings. Others may say "well what about the life that you have in your body, warm blood running in your veins, how could you say something so ridiculous about yourself like that? Can't you express yourself about any other issue rather than your Tourette's. Look hear, I will not apologize for the high self-esteem that I have now, for loving myself unconditionally which I should've developed a prognosis way earlier in my young childhood years.

I will not apologize for the new me speaking and expressing my mind, saying what I feel, taking action towards life and all things in general. I have changed in a way that leaves me flabbergasted when I look back and see how I have developed and have transformed from being this little nobody who was locked up inside a treacherous being called, "Me" into a new person!

But what I will apologize for is all of the attitudes and bitterness, the vulgarity of my language that I used and said towards anyone and everyone that I snapped on out loud or under my breathe, and for all of the uncontrollable ugly behavior I've bestowed and lashed out on you such a long time ago, "I am sorry"

Please know this, I was a young kid growing up in the early 80's and 90's in the State of Connecticut with bad shadows. Living in a very ghostly transitional time zone left with despair 90% of my life. I had and still have a disability!

No father for me or my brother (we have 2 different dads) God Bless him wherever he may be at and I look forward to the day that we will meet, if he is still alive.

So I had to take on the responsibility of various roles in my little brother's life that could help benefit some or all of the absent bodies that were not present or were present, but haven't been around a beautiful being who is and has been well adjusted now without those that were ignorant in behavior enough to skip out on life, a son, sons that are doing just fine now!!

Not because of the money or materialistic things that have been restored to each of it's rightful owner, but because of the lack thereof, the poorness, despair, hatred and hurt that has now been wiped clean by God's smooth grace. Every character role model in my life that was lost or was lost semi-partially, temporarily, or never has been filled, replaced, and restored by Gods own way.

Like being a good friend, a big brother, a father figure in some ways or another, an uncle or grandfather, a friend from the streets, a teacher, I try to fill the different male role category as best as I know how and try to be exclusive in my brother's life as much as possible.

Trying to be a positive role model for him that's another story. You guys might say "well you said it yourself on bridging some of the gaps missing from home in a family mode. How is being a positive role model a different scenario from those sequences?? My life definition of a positive role model is God! He is someone who is always and will always be there no matter what you do and go through. The only thing is you cannot see Him with your eyes physically, but you can sense him emotionally, spiritually, mentally, physically inward or outwardly. He is everywhere.

A positive role model I am not!! Not for my brother, or anyone else that may see me as one. And if you stepped to me and ask me if I can be your role model? I'd say "no never that, sorry can't do it. So don't ask! Because I don't want to be, it's not in me or my nature. After a lot of the things that I have done and/or did personally and still do in some ways or another, it is way too much work.

Even though my kid sib looks up to me (Yo son I appreciate that from the bottom of my heart)

Being beaten, stepped on, put down by many, not revealing my emotions. Staying closed-up behind a wall stenched in my own sour stale shell that kept me bound inside a black hole. Leading to a place full of sorrow trapped in carelessness to a point, as if I wanted absolutely nothing more than to give up on anything and everything that I could ever do or ever get my hands on.

My body was like a human recycling piggy bank safe at a bank with a shooting range built together or in laymen's terms "a walking, talking time bomb", Tic tic boom! Ha, nobody was safe from me and/or around me, for real.

You could deposit harsh feelings, negative energy, drama, or whatever. In return, I would shoot back my anger at you like weapons of mass destruction.

I'd load up all of my ammo from my chest, heart and brain. My chest stored up all of the mad fuel that builds up, then deposited straight into my heart, which pumps the mad fuel dwelling from head to toe deep within.

Hidden behind a bright smile, nice character, respectable, decent, mannerable young fella, you'd never guessed during a calm debate you would get to see and know the flip side, you didn't know that I would express everything hurting inside me once I got mad. Issues get so high at times to where anything and everything was targeted. Each time I would load up the ammo stored inside of my chest that I had, and fire it right back at you in many ways possible.

I let everything build up then release it manly at my mom's who was one of my main targets. which wasn't right at all because half the time she never knew what was going on unless I reacted outwardly. She didn't like the attitudes or moods swings. You say one little thing to me and boom I implode, explode, and then I feel better. I really didn't know how to express my true feelings right then and there when someone would upset me, I'd accept the bull crap but wouldn't give it back. "Not no more!" Like my man Havoc say "We can get it on if the drama or beef occurs, Yo I'm a cool ass dude til you push me sir! That verse is from Amerikaz Nightmare Very Big Ups to Havoc & Prodigy of Mobb Deep A Dynamic Duo by the way who's still pioneering the music game peace yall.

Back to the subject. I really don't blow-up-chuate anymore. My Tourette Syndrome has given me so many different experiences in life from getting whiplashed and punished by my mom's. In ways that was well above average to any other kids my age receiving beatings from their parents. No matter how much trouble any kid got into it could not compare to my ranks. I got beat a lot like Forrest Gump "I got whooped uh-la!

On the upside, females would approach me and say that my Tourette's is cool, it made me cute or they just liked the way I move, jump, jerk, shake and make noise. Who knew? That having a medical condition is an A+ with some of the females!! To me it's kinda strange, but it boosted my self-esteem tremendously. I'll speak for all guys in the disability field by saying that a disability enhances or heightens a female's smitten interest towards us, at least I think it does?

I was taken a medication called Haloperidol (haldol for short)…It was supposed to help my twitching mode calm down maybe slow up the condition. No results, only side affects, so I smoked weed?? You heard me right. Weed, Pot, Mary Jane, Trees, Grass, Herbal Essence, Purple Haze, Sticky Icky, Hydro, Popeye's Spinach, Green, Trizz, Budd Boo-dah lova's everywhere whatever you callin it, yaw know what I mean.

It helped in ways those stupid pills couldn't. Understand that Chapter 1 may seem like the introduction but it's not, I don't really know how to piece a book together but I'm trying though bare wit me. I am showing yall a pre-background basis of Me, Myself, and My Tourette Syndrome has meant to 1 another.

Several years ago was when I stepped outta high school. I graduated from Pearl-Cohn with a Special-Ed Diploma, "I am very proud of myself for even getting one". My freshmen year was pure Hell!! Just moved away from home (Connecticut) into a totally new State (Tennessee)…I made several trips to Tennessee with my Grandparents, my moms, my lil brother, my uncle and several church folks. All my life I've traveled. We moved around a lot.

I loved to travel, traveling to me is being free, roaming and never staying put where you are currently at. Aint No Limit to where I's going, I'd go plum crazy if I'd just permanently stayed where I was at. I will always love my home team always. Call me Dorky instead of Dorothy when she say "there's no place like home," "there's no place well you get what I saying right.

When we moved Out of State it was from CT (Connecticut) it looks like an Iron skillet so does Massachusetts, our States are like fraternal twins. God told my mom's to move, so we did!

Obedience is a keen sense to deal with God "Just Do It" I didn't question God or mom's, you can abort what your mom or any other human being might say unless It's God flowing through them to tell you something but you Do Not Abort GOD when he talks to you. I didn't get upset, raise hell, worry about persons, places or things or nothing like that. We sold everything we had in the house for extra money, packed up what we weren't going to take and left it in the basement of our 3 family home.

A 3 family home is a tall house with 3 different floors stacked on top of one another connected with balcony's attached front and back. There're really nice, they give great views, very relaxing one word for'em WOW!

Everyone has balcony's, So if you move into one or you see or know somebody with one they have what there neighbors have, because it balances out the whole building. You can't have one balcony and the other 2 floors not have one it won't look right at all. Take my word for it and just move into a 3 story family house and you will see what I'm talking about.

Up there it is colonial like, there are more 2 & 3 families houses all over the place not just in certain areas whether good or bad, it's nice everywhere I really mean it.

We packed our Sentra lightly with just enough things to get us by till we reed-up for the long road trip we'd have to endure to Tennessee. We moved to Knoxville Tennessee, for about a year then packed and threw stuff away, the usual routine for us "mission type people."

Then, we moved again this time to Nashville, Tennessee. My mom had gotten a job at our "former church headquarters" where we are no longer members, so we moved.

On the road again, I swear I feel like one of God's groupies the way we move! We stayed in Nashville in a fairly decent area. We lived a short period in these dorms (1 room with two beds, a small refrigerator, but no place to cook) that "our former church" owned that we used to attend. Mom's and I worked for them for awhile. She was one of the receptionist/typist and I worked with the older men doing maintenance, carpentry, janitorial, landscaping, etc.

In 95' I became the "new kid on the block," the new kid with Tourette's. I knew people from church but not from the streets yet. I only knew one female in the entire school from "my former church." My high school was in a pretty rough neighborhood with friends surviving the game by all means necessary. "Big-Up's to those of you at Pearl-Cohn from my heart to yours, 1 Luv!! Holla!" I'll see you soon.

I wanted to dropout 6 months early on into my freshman status. I went through some craziness, but through it all I overcame, I saw, I graduated with a Special-Ed Diploma.

People, "Don't let anyone! And I mean No one!" tell you what you can or cannot do with your life, especially when they're not doing anything with their lives. You can still make it in this world without the credentials of diplomas, degrees, awards, certificates, or any other type of goal setting paper status.

There are a lot of people who have dropped out of and/or never went to school who have become successful in some ways or another. GED's or Special-Ed Diplomas such as myself, it doesn't matter "YOU CAN STILL SURVIVE and SUCCEED, I DID, LOOK AT ME NOW!!!"

Just keep reading on yall, I aint done yet.

2

The age of 7 was when I first became diagnosed with my lovely companion, Tourette's Syndrome. I say that about it because I really do Love It! 17 years ago, I couldn't vibe with you about this. If you were to ask me how I felt about my condition, I would never say that I love or accepted it, I hated it! But now, man please, I express myself openly.

In scientific studies, the definition of Tourette Syndrome is a neurological disorder characterized by involuntary body movements (tics) "not the blood sucking flesh imbedding bugs", and uncontrollable vocal sounds.

In a minority of cases, the vocalizations can include socially inappropriate words and phrases called coprolalia. The outbursts are neither intentional nor purposeful. The involuntary symptoms can include eye blinking, repetitive throat clearing, sniffing, stuttering sentences, arm thrusting, kicking movements, shoulder shrugging, jumping, head twitching, grabbing or tugging of oneself, cussing involuntarily, unwanted or bothersome thoughts, ritualistic behaviors, limited facial expressions, and many other forms that I don't know about yet.

These and all other symptoms typically appear before the age of 18 and the condition occurs in all ethnic groups with males becoming affected 3 to 4 times more likely to receive TS than females. Although the symptoms of TS vary from person to person and range from very mild to severe, the majority of cases fall into the mild category. Associated conditions can include intentional problems, impulsiveness and learning disabilities.

Most people with Ts lead productive lives and participate in all professions. Increased public understanding and tolerance of TS symptoms are of paramount importance to people with Tourette Syndrome

The disorder Tourette Syndrome that I, along with so many other people have had, and/or will have in the near future was named for a French neuropsychiatrist who successfully assessed the disorder in the late 1800s: His name is Georges

Gilles de la Tourette (born Georges Albert Edouard Brutus Gilles de la Tourette!)…In 1857, he made several valuable contributions to medicine and literature. His greatest achievements were in the studies of hysteria and hypnotism; a competent neuropsychiatrist, who was particularly interested in therapy. With a fellow colleague, he wrote a highly perceptive analysis of Sister Jeanne des Agnes' account of her "hysterical illness" which was caused by her unrequited love for a priest.

Here are a few more historical examples of everyday people who became famous or turned celebrity that had Tourette Syndrome and did not let their medical condition or stupid, ignorant lame individuals stop them from wanting and becoming very successful in life.

On a personal note of mine, to all of you dead, negative, lifeless haters who are a wastes of God's human creation, "I am talking to You!" each and every single one of you maggots that doubted behind our backs, in front of our faces, under your breathe, or to others that my brother, mother, me and anybody else that was or is trying to make and be something with themselves.

These people as well as I are prime examples who have made something with our lives from a disabled state of mind.

From (1756-1791) Wolfgang Amadeus Mozart, the famous piano player musician had the disorder of Tourette Syndrome, who cut off the folks and drama that was plagued around him and transisted into a classical revolutionaries as an artist, who's musical masterpieces are still heared and listened too, played and performed by people world wide today as we speak.

Myles R, Walker (Me), author, rapper, drummer, poet, writer, and activist, etc.

So you see, this disability hasn't become some newfound latest discovery in Science. This TS case of research has been around way over a century or more maybe even earlier I don't know.

Researchers have not developed a cure for it yet, will they ever find a cure for TS and everything affiliated with it?? Who knows? Only God and time will tell, that's all I can say. As far as more TS studies go, information keeps on rollin, and there is still a great deal about TS that scientist, researchers, and people don't know about.

Want to know more about Tourette Syndrome, just go to any library available to dig up any information on TS from the computer and its numerous websites, the archives machine, numerous books, newspapers, and other written and/or printed legislative documentation. Log onto: ts@tsa-usa.org or http://www.tsa-usa.org

I hope that you will gain more wisdom, knowledge, understanding and study up on Tourette Syndrome and may your horizons be broadened.

3

Noises, weird sounds, and gibberish started to develop just like the TS definition explained in previous articles that I've read. I wasn't prepared in any way, shape form, or fashion of any kind for what was once a light twitching nightmare now going to become a Living Hell of Reality.

It scared me and made me feel like one of those fictional stories we see, watch, and hear about from the newspapers, books, television shows and movies etc...Like the Lockness monster, Big Foot, The Abominable Snowman, Aliens, Vampires, Ghouls-N-Ghost, Moby Dick, you know all them type stories. Let me break it down for you. Tourette's is just like these fictional stories that we've encountered way back when, but with the exception that TS stories are not fiction.

The facts have much depth to its origin which has made some reviews in history dating back beyond a century. So it's not like people are just noticing what it is, although many years ago nobody knew what TS was. "I'm just trying to drop a Lil science folks"

Anyway, I'm gaining involuntary reactions from my throat, conjoining with my diaphragm (F.Y.I; Diaphragm helps give people who sing stronger notes ditto with my TS)...TS is constantly evolving never prone to stay the same. Animals I saw outside, at the zoo, on the discovery channel or wherever, I'd imitate. Some of those imitations caught up with me. Dig this? I could laugh and yelp like Hyenas or spider monkeys, bark like dogs, black crows, cars that had performance mufflers, whistles, bells and sirens, when I'd talk my sentences would get repetitive with slurred up with stuttering,

When I walked, I would shuffle my feet forward causing the tread in the forefoot of my shoes to wear down quicker than a most life spans in sneakers, I skipped, hopped and jumped all at once. Many quarks developed and changed, sometimes I thought my quarks would switch every 3 months like the 4 seasons of Winter, Spring, Summer and Fall. Sound among sounds, jerks, quarks, gibberish, new involuntary movements etc. My condition had more cycles in 1 year than any female having her monthly period with P.M.S. and a side of menopausal mood swings.

This medical condition I was experiencing wasn't some walk in the park. This, this mode of mechanics was about to ruin my life forever, so I thought. It did ruin my childhood in some ways because I started feeling depressed, getting anxiety attacks, social anxiety attacks that left me not wanting to do anything and be around anyone which kept me bound from many opportunities.

People, we know when we are sick, hurt, depressed, not loved, are being abused in some form, so what do we do?? We take the proper precautions to deal with whatever is bothering us. I didn't know that they had special facilities and services that handle the caring requirements of Tourette Syndrome.

That is why we can't get upset when something goes wrong, we should rejoice and be glad in it and not get upset. When you get frustrated it won't solve anything, it'll make what you're going through a lot worse if you don't trust, believe, and have faith in God. Remember that faith without works is dead; we can't sit back and rely on him to do everything. Nope! We gotta do something too.

Have <u>Faith</u>, <u>Trust</u>, & <u>Believe In GOD </u>and <u>Believe in </u>Yourself which is the Truest Motto In Life Itself!!

4

Months have gone by my body is jumping in one direction and my voice is sounding off in another. Put those two factors together and you got yourself a human jackhammer with a built in keyboard beat machine. My Tourette's was like a light switch you flick on and off. Between the ages of 7 and 8 my TS began to play games with me. Rapidly disappearing completely for a month or so, comeback and stay for another month, then once again go away.

For a year and a half, it continuously played games with me, and I never ever knew that it could do that. A triple take side show was in affect, like a circus, the funny freak, the freak show, and haunted house all combined into one; so to speak.

[1] Like any great circus popping threw town. It would create a buzz and let everyone know that there is a show in town.

[2] The freak show would gather up all of the unwanted attention for all to see something unique, original, and not ever seen in the ordinary.

[3] The Funny Freak Show as you all know of course would provide the humor for the upcoming event in amusing the people making them people laugh hysterically. And finally last but certainly not least of this attracting rendition, the fourth and final part of the closing adventure;

[4] The Haunted House had all the scary sounds and creepy moves that fascinated and freaked people out.

You might understand what I have just explained in my little world of vision, but that is what my episode felt like at the time.

Was I hallucinating, is this a bad dream or nightmare, could Tourette Syndrome really do such a thing as this. I wonder if other individuals have experienced some, any or all of the same scenarios with TS that I've regulated. They may or may not have, I just hope that each and every single one you who have similar episodes of various TS issues and/or any other type of disability. Talk about it and do not keep it bottled up inside, go get help and get it out there cause it could save someone else's life who may think about committing suicide or a violent act.

Help save someone who isn't as fortunate as you might be in life. I was always taught to help and not be selfish. What you make happen for someone else, can happen for you. It is so vital that we help someone who doesn't receive any Love and support from family, friends, the church. It is mandatory for churches to help the world, not the government.

The government isn't responsible for what goes on in the streets. The church is supposed to be the support system for the fatherless, strangers, orphans, widows, children and the poor and all who need help and TLC services.

But some don't do it, "Believe me, I know I've been in this same predicament". Me and my 2 family members can testify to that. To this very day, grudges, rejection and lost love are still held against us this very present day and time that we liven in right know. It's been so many years ago and people who know who they are, are still acting grimy.

But its okay, because I have Loved, Forgiven and Forgotten each and every single one of you for your cruel intentions in prayer." Thank You Very Much Sincerely!!. No hatred here by a long shot. **Peace 5,000!!!**

5

My mom's gave me many beatings and put me on punishment day in and day out for my condition because she thought that I was just spazzed out. "Yes Yes Yall", I got handled everyday (seriously) no joke "she had it in for me".

My teachers could call my moms at work or home and tell her that I'm the only kid in the world who has ever made the straightest A's in the entire State of Connecticut, and she would still beat for spazzen out no matter what good thing I did, the beatings kept on coming and coming.

Anytime and every time that she felt like it she'd grab something left or right. Switches, belts, ironing cords, extension cords, her hands, shoes, my brother and I pool sticks. I aint exaggerating either, anything handy enough that could be used as a beating utensil was surely used.

There was not a day that didn't go by without a whip lashed moment. I knew something was wrong with me but she didn't know that. To all of you asking the questions; "Do you Love your Mamma really good? **Yes!** Are you holding back any pain or aggression towards her for beating you excessively the way that she did. **No!**...To this day we can still laugh and joke about that and other crazy things that have happened to us and still feel free.

"Tell em' Ma"....

Back then, I guess I was really young and stupid and I really didn't know what I was doing in raising children (Myles, I need to take the time again which I certainly don't mind telling you that I am truly sorry for the beatings that you received and I never meant to hurt you, I LOVE YOU AND YOUR BROTHER ROBERT WITH ALL OF MY HEART, I WOULD NOT INTENTIONALLY DO ANYTHING TO HURT YOU AND YOUR BROTHER. I AM TRULY SORRY, AND I ASK FOR YOUR FORGIVENESS AS I HAVE ALREADY DONE, BUT I DON'T MIND SAYING IT AGAIN AND AGAIN! YOU AND YOUR BROTHER, ARE A VERY SPECIAL PART OF

MY LIFE (GOD AND JESUS IS FIRST AND THEN YOU AND YOUR BROTHER COME IN SECOND!

YOU ARE BOTH GOD FEARING, WONDERFUL, KIND, HAND-SOME, LOVING, INTELLIGENT, SUCCESSFUL MEN, AND I THANK GOD FOR BOTH OF YOU EVERY SINGLE DAY!! NOT JUST SAYING THESE THINGS ON PAPER, BUT I SAY THEM TO YOU EVERY DAY SOMETIMES TWO OR MORE TIMES A DAY!! GOD HAS BLESSED ME WITH TWO MEN WHO I AM VERY PROUD OF!! GOD HAS BLESSED ME TO BE YOUR MOTHER AND BY THAT I AM HONOURED!!

We had been through so many things together, I sometimes thought that I was right in most things, but in whipping you (Robert received whippings as well) it did not make it right especially when you had a medical condition.

I though that you were just trying to get attention, but then when the Doctor told me that you had Tourette Syndrome which I had never heard of, I was in total denial, because I did not want to believe that there was something wrong with my child.

I HAVE NEVER ONCE BEEN ASHAMED OF YOU, I AM AND ALWAYS WILL BE PROUD OF YOU AND YOUR BROTHER ROBERT YOU BOTH ARE GOOD MEN!!!!

I am glad that you have forgiven me for not knowing how to raise a son with Tourette Syndrome, but I have learned through trial and error and especially by my Faith in God! You had 23 years of seeing the good and the bad side of parent-ing, but I THANK GOD THAT I HAVE LEARNED THE RIGHT WAY TO GO AND TO TRY AND RAISE YOU AND YOUR BROTHER ROBERT IN A GOD FEARING MANNER!

Having a son with a medical condition is not easy for any parent, especially a single mother, but we have made it and we are making it with God's Help!!!

I know that I am sometimes too protective of you and your brother, because I did not want you both to be hurt, but I know now that God will protect and take care of both of you! I asked God to help me raise you both and I thank God that

I listened to him and changed my life around! I LOVE YOU BOTH!!!!! ALWAYS!!!

MA, I <u>LOVE YOU</u>, ROBERT <u>LOVE'S YOU</u>, AND We BOTH <u>LOVE YOU</u> WITH ALL OF OUR HEARTS!!

ILUV WARRIOR GLORIA

Being lonely sometimes, can have it's disadvantages when you are solo or by yourself. You want someone to love and show affection too, a companion who will share life with you in every aspect possible, someone that can trade constant smiles, laughter, happy and sad feelings. Emotions overwhelmed with joy every time you see one another's face your cherishing each moment as if it were you very last. We'll that is what I felt for the first time when I laid eyes on such a beautiful, innocent, being…*MY BROTHER Robert (Frogge/Skillet Head)*

$SIKE$

HA!! HA!! HA!! Hardy HAR HAR HAR. None of yall saw that coming did you?? Nope, no you didn't tella truth. I gotcha good with dat romantic swing swing and had you thinking that I was talking about some shorty from way back.

I bet that a lot of you females I once knew and got rejected by thought that I was aiming at you in the paragraph above this one. "Sorry I wasn't" I am talking bout my baby boy brother Frogge. I wonder whatcha faces look like right about now.

Again, I am talking about **MY SON, MY BROTHER, MY FRIEND TO THE END, ROBERT,** the one That I raised after he was born and for 16 years and still counting. The one that I asked, prayed, and wanted God to send to me when I was lonely, when I needed a companion in life, a playmate that would love me for me no matter what. Guess what?? He's been growing with me since he was a seed.

Even though I have a medical condition, he never once was ashamed of me, never put me down or made me feel low. My Tourette's doesn't bother him and never has, he won't even make fun of me even if I ask him too. He be like "naw that's not funny, "I aint gonna do that".

People that I know, will rank on me instantly, more than Frogge will, and have a ball doing it. But as far as Frogge goes, he might slide a rank in here or there once in a blue moon, if he feels like doing it

He always tried to build me up and help me out with whatever it is or was that I needed help and/or support with. We've done a lot of stuff together and still do. We have and collect toys of all kinds, we wrestle and fight one another, call each other all kinda names, we spend the night in each others rooms just like friends do. I cook for him and he cook's for me, we stick up and stick by each other, working out, hanging out in the streets from A to Z, we huddle together.

He's my Big Brother and I am his Little Brother, It's crazy nah mean. that's how we see each other most times now-a-days. Since he's gotten a lot older in age and more grown up mentally, He no longer sports the shadow of a little brother anymore "I do, I sport the little brother shadow"

Yo Son talk to em',

Hi my name is Robert Hill and I am 16 years old and my brother Myles has a condition called Tourette Syndrome. He's had it ever since he was little. He's is cool and a good friend and a brother, but most importantly he is like a father to me. He raised me ever since I came out my mothers stomach. He does almost every thing for me, and if I wanted to go some where he can talk my mother into it. People that know him tell me all the time that he is cool and they wish that they had a brother like that. I really like to go places with him, some people would think that it would faze me, people always stare, but it doesn't faze me at all. **I love my brother very much you would too if you knew him!!**

6

"In Denial or Living a Lie, What does that phrase mean?? Are you or could you be that person? Do you know someone like that? I know someone like that yall. (Pause) "You do?" "Yes! Yes! Yall I Do!" Who is it???>>>> ME! What do you mean You??

"Look at you gossiping folks ready and waiting to here the skinny about me"

I used to be "in denial or live a lie" when I was just a lad. "Oh Yeah", On the days that I was appointed on to go see my doctor, I would prepare myself for **T.I.C. Stealth Mode**. A mode that **transforms** your attitude, feelings and behavior patterns about TS, into an **invisible character**.

In laymen's terms, I would reject my true self and keep him hostage whenever I had to express how I felt having TS and what was wrong and/or bothering me. "Ah!!, those laymen's terms was long wasn't they?". I'd switch my behavior from, "I Feel Good", to, "Get Off My Chest" which is not a good way to waste your time denying and lying to whomever your physician is.

Because I really believe that when doctors take notes and learn from you, they record the info into a study that will help elaborate futuristic prognosis's for others that have the same likeness and/or familiarity in the medical condition we posses, in order to help someone else who deals with the same thing.

I bottled up everything like **Very Fine Apple Juice**. "I'm very fine thank you for asking," but I'm not sharing my apples with you". It does nothing but shred you all inside.

Real Men Cry, Real Men emotionally express themselves, Real Men blow off steam orally. It took me along time to shed my skin. You know the saying "I wear my feelings on my arms", that was me as a prime example. Nothing had changed for me whenever I went to see the doctor.

They already knew what was up with me just by observing the fake blanket hovering over my real self. People let me tell you from experience, "Do Not! I repeat, Do Not! Ball up your emotions inside yourself and keep them hidden. Go talk to someone who can help you, get them out early. Any time something's wrong find an activity that'll absorb your stressful tensions.

God Bless Dr. Kleinman who is a Pediatric Neurologist, who loved, cared for, and tried to help me the best way possible even though I'd reneged all of her questions that had everything to do with my Tourette's and well being.

7

This is going to take awhile of what I am about to say. To me it seems like a poem that went graphically haywire in my cerebral cortex. "I don't know in what way or how you are going to react to this". Maybe you'll have an eyegasm by the time you finish reading it.

These are my thoughts and perspectives on I had flowin threw my head about what high school was gonna be like for me. "Oh Yeah, one more thing", I gotta lotta commas and question marks everywhere…(Check me out)

When I became fresh meat I was in for a lot of up's and downs, drama, young adolescence setting in, you know what anybody dreads about in high school. The aphrodisiac of a young kid making a switch to early adulthood. Being around older peers, the peer pressure's of sex, drugs, and teenager pregnancy, trying to fit in with different groups of kids as far as style like punk, skate, preppy, smart, dum, leaders, followers, jocks, rock-n-roll, religious, good, bad, racial aliens, sexual gender preference.

What activities are pursued for after school projects by kids. Could it be sports, baseball, basketball, football, track and field. Swimming, volleyball, soccer, gymnastics, chorus, tutoring or getting tutored from a teacher or one another. Being a mentor to someone that needs a positive re-enforcer. Helping grade papers or organize paper work that will be essential throughout the week.

Does anyone hangout with each other after school? Where do they go and what do they do? Ride bikes, hanging at the mall, hanging on the block just chillin, or huggin the block hustling. Playing video games or sports, listening to music or making a band, watching movies or studying at school or at someone's house spending the night. Doing volunteer work for a business and/or helping an individual around their house doing whatever daily chores necessary. Getting paid by the hour at a real job. Having sex, masturbating or having no sex at all which is safer.

There are a lot of clubs that are available to join? As far as band chorus, some sort of glee club, chess club, arts and/or crafts club, boys or girls scouts club, band, dance club, half-timers, auto mechanics, shop class, step class, etc. There are a lot clubs to participate in. Pardon me for leaving out any other clubs that I've forgotten to mention.

So many people gathered together on an everyday, day to day basis, 5 days a week in one huge facility trying to get to know you. Many questions, answers and other things to learn about you, yourself, your fellow peers and the faculty members around you.

Remember the old saying of how curiosity killed the cat, well what kind of curiosity floating in the atmosphere that maybe you or someone around you could be thinking about you or the next persons, concerning sexual preference. Is he or she heterosexual, gay, homosexual, bisexual, transsexual, trysexual, homophobic, transvestite, hermaphrodite, or object?

Who's having sex? Who's a virgin and saving themselves?, Who doesn't want to be a virgin and wants to be devirginized? Who's been with 1 or more partners.

Don't sit their and front like **YOU** aint never pondered these things in your head before.

Answer these 2 questions then. Who's real and who's fake? What's real and what's fake? **Real** and **Fake,** what do these two words mean to you in your everyday life? These two words are scattered, used and found everywhere. God is real, real love, life and Death is real. **Real** can even turn into fake. **Fake** people, fake breast, fake stories, fake feelings and emotions. Real and fake can be with you at home, work, school, church, and/or found within yourself.

Schools and churches are in some ways similar to each other. The preacher is like the main principal, the ushers and deacons are like the school board faculty members, the congregation of people can vary from small to large. The teachers and students huddle into classrooms just like Sunday School on Sunday's

People of all individual races and religions come together to learn, whether they're Christians, atheist, Baptist, Pentecostal, Jewish, Mormon, Buddhist,

Islamic, Muslim, K K K, skinhead, redneck, rebel, communist, Arabic or Egyptian, believer or nonbeliever.

All of that doesn't matter anyway because **WE ARE ALL 1 Nation Under GOD!!**

Again with the Real or Fake, Love vs. Hate, battle of the sexes between the dominant male and female genders of whose stronger. Who is handicapped, disabled, scarred, burned, scorned, and/or has a physical deformity or amputated body parts. Who comes from a dysfunctional family?

Who has a sexual transmitting disease? Who is or could be pregnant? Who's selling or using drugs? Who's packing or bringing guns and knives to school?, Which students have a rap sheet as far as being in or out of juvenile hall or jail?, Who and where are the bullies if they're any, and why are they punking out others? Which kids need help?

"Hey you guys!!" Teachers of all kinds aint gonna feel me on this one."

I was even skeptical about the teachers, "you know?" Despite having Tourette's I wondered if the teachers cared about me as they claim. I had or was put into special classes more than regular classes. I wanted to be placed with the kids who got taught a bolder curriculum than I. By the age 10 and up, my TS was really full blown meaning (it grew and glued itself to me permanently)...I didn't like it but I had to deal with it.

I fought for myself and my mom's fought for me in trying to get me into regular classes, but I was still forced beyond my will. Every new school year I would apply for regular classes like social studies 1, geometry or whatever, but to no avail once I got my hands on my new schedule it would read special-ed this or special-ed that. I know for a fact that alot of my classes were whack, did they give me a chance, Nope! They just shoved me in the attic to collect dust and spider webs.

They were way to critical about my well being in the classroom at least I thought so. Everyday I'd worry about getting kicked outta class over TS?? I still wonder about all my teachers, **did they really mind putting up with my Tourette's??**

Will I be denied to work? Will I disturb the students? Will I be able to work or will my twitching keep me so jumpy that it'll affect my ability to work? Will I be removed from class and be excluded from group projects? Will the teachers find some way to get rid of me just because they get frustrated and the barking-N-yellping noises (they can't stop it though). Will I be placed with other kids who have special needs and interests which never ever bothered me at all, because at least I knew that I was in a comfortable area with teachers who loved to work with the disabled kids. Or do they really love us?? hmmm?? A lot of things rambled on inside my head. On a day to day basis I tried to prepare myself for the worse beforehand, so that it wouldn't make me as agitated as usual.

People, parents, teachers, friends, neighbors, family members, this is the reason why that I am drawing your attention towards this matter. If you know a disabled individual(s) that wants to be in regular or stronger classes, help them to achieve and succeed in doing so. **"Fight! Help, standby, and believe in those that don't believe in themselves.**

"Please don't rob that person of his or her individual rights for wanting to better themselves. If they want to be in regular classes "let them." It'll make a great difference and change the ways and minds of alot of people that don't have faith enough to pull through a struggle.

How many times must I say or repeat myself. Start a coalition, a program, a foundation, or corporation that will give students in school hope of a better future at hand. Whatever it takes to make footprints leading towards a better life. You wouldn't want someone else to reject or deny your child the right of passage in regular classes, "now would you??"

Everyday, we should take time out to Thank God. Stop and smell the roses, feed, cloth, love, provide and help someone in need, sow Seeds. Care for a stray animal, learn something new by the second, let not life pass you or someone else by. Motivate and regulate, don't be fruitful and multiply if you can't function your own humanities. Grow a plant into a dream, use what you have wisely and make it greater.

It's cool now because I still made it outta school period, with TS and a Special-Ed diploma. **"So laugh now or forever holds your peace."**

8

Alrighty then, I am just about finished with this book. So bare with me as we go through these few Chapters or so, which I don't exactly know how long each Chapter is going to be, that's why I'm talking to you about this, because I want to at least take up some space on this one.

For a long time I was taking some prescription drug called "Haloperidol, or Haldol for short"…I first took this medicine between the ages of 10 or 11. I took it off and on for 4 ½ years. Haloperidol is a medication that is prescribed for people who have a mental illness, "I don't have a mental illness", "I'm mad now yall fa real".

The only thing that I've had and still have on earth in life to this very day is God and Tourette Syndrome. All of the years that have gone and passed by, I'm up here taking pills I that are totally irrelevant towards my condition, besides the fact of me being a young kid, "I didn't know, nor did my mother"…

Crazy as this may sound, about a year and a half ago, I was watching TV. And I remember these news reports about the various problems and concerns about a certain SUV.

Well, one evening I was watching Dateline, and the Journalist Stone Phillips, along with several other journalists were interviewing numerous people about their street accident they've encountered with their SUV's. There was one particular African-American married couple being interviewed.

They had been in a car accident at the time. When the camera zoomed in on the wife, she caught my attention when she spoke about the medication the doctors prescribed for her to take upon her get well status. And one of the most fascinating paragraphs that she said, "have stuck with me since that time". She said that her doctors and I quote, that "she was given a prescription drug called Haloperidol or Haldol for short"

A medication that is only and I repeat, only supposed to be prescribed and given to patients who are mentally ill and/or are developing symptoms of mental illness. She was prescribed the wrong medication; she wasn't supposed to get Haldol. Nobody should be recommended to take a medication that is not fit for their individual purpose, let alone a car accident.

"I was flabbergasted with Ripley's Believe it or Not Emotions fa Real!! When I heard that, I emecheitly (slang for immediately) turned the tube up. I have TS, but she doesn't and we don't know each other on top of that. Mrs. Lady being interviewed by Dateline,"

Thank You Very Much for that knowledgeable information that you've said publicly for the entire world and individuals with TS to see, hear, and know about. **Thank You!!** All this time has gone by and I didn't do any research on the vital issue.

Weed helped me and my Tourette's better than those pills could in the physical sense of medication. Mary Jane kept me at bay.

For those of you who are asking this question in your head or out loud. "Yes I do know the side affects of weed, all medicines have or may have side affects to them. Whether its Alka-Seltzer to Zanax "I'm not stupid" You thought that I was going to leave that part out didn't you.

I telling you guys this because I simply want you guys to know what it was like for me when I smoked weed. "You heard me right, I aint ssst, ssst, ssst, stutter folks". **My cries 2 tears in a bucket it, bump It, let's take it too the stage.**

If you don't have Tourette Syndrome, but you may have a certain type of medical condition or not, gain some knowledge, talk to your Doctor, and take necessary actions with medication.

After the diagnostically studies and tests were done on me and my Tourette Syndrome, my doctor determined what medication I was going to take. The pills I took I had to take ingestionally before or after I ate.

The colors were orange and white I believe. The instructions that my doctor gave me on taking were stamped on the front of the bottle just like any other medication you take. It didn't have any nasty or bitter tastes to it that would make squint my eyes. They were no bigger than the size of popcorn kernel.

One time, I went to an organic store and got some of these fun dissolving pills that you put under your tongue. The doctor who offered a recommendation about those whack pills thought that they could help me if I try them. This person wasn't my normal go-see, and didn't know what they were talking about.

My mother and I went to the organic store and purchased them, We got em' we left, and as soon as we got in the car I took two and placed em' under my tongue just like the directions said so. For a month or so I did follow this weak process 3 times a day, I didn't see or feel any gradual responses, so I stopped taking them end of story.

The pills directions would change sometimes depending on the severity of my condition meaning, if my TS would act up or not seem like it would slow down or get any calmer, than my dosage (the milligrams escalate higher) would upgrade strongly to maybe help or correct the energy and/or intensity of my TS whenever my movements became a little over board.

Again, at other times my dosage (the milligrams escalate lower) would down grade if my TS's energy was level or stable to where didn't need extra milligrams in my pills. My instructions were to take the pills 1 ½ in the morning, 2 in the afternoon, and 1 in the evening before I go Nite-Nite.

Sometimes I wouldn't even take it at all; I'd go the whole 24hrs without taking my medications. Many times my mother would stand in front of me, and watch me with her own two eyes, just to make sure that I do the right thing.

Another way of her so called "I-Spy checkmate moves", is scanning my refill bottles to see if pills were decreasing daily. The simplicity of taking my medication was futile to her, but not for me "Ah-uh"

It either went in the trash, flushed down the toilet or sink, thrown outta the window, stepped on, sucked up by the vacuum cleaner, or disposed of by any other means necessary. As long as I could do away wit it and not have to deal wit it I was cool.

So one day, I was chillin, in the somewhere in between the year of 95', I can't really remember the month or day, but it was the very last day for those jerk pills. I got fed up with it and gave my mother an ultimatum. I was no longer going to take my medicine, and if she didn't like it, then she could beat me all over again. But I didn't care one bit, all's I knew **"No More"**

I usually never ever felt any different after those pills were in my system. Most of the time I would just feel the same way I did before, and for the most part, I contracted side affects. My hands would shake a lot, I couldn't focus on different tasks at hand, and I had no facial expressions for the camera or anyone that wanted to see me smile. I never knew that facial expressions of person with TS were hindered or not shown enough voluntarily by someone with Tics. Maybe that's why I don't smile a lot.

Almost every single picture that I've had snapped by a professional photographer, shows me ice grillin, mean muggin. I looked like I'm wasn't happy, faking smiles with a smerk in front of it all because of my lack of happiness that I've experienced for so long. What I'm tryin to say is that my TS tends to bully my facial expressions.

Some things have changed and over the years that I've been rehabilitating myself, my attitude, they way I look at the world an other people, and try to reincarnate different things, journeys, and experiences that was held back from within myself.

9

In Chapter 8 I told you guys about the pills that I was taken, what they did or was supposed do for me. And I also told you about Mary Jane (weed) and what she did for me that the pills couldn't do. I didn't know that marijuana is or can be prescribed to individual(s) with Tourette Sydrome.

When I heard that, I started reading information, watching documentaries and I talked to a lot of doctors, pharmacist, and other people who could inform me about some of the questions and answers that I had concerning this matter.

Yes I know what your saying right about know, "But you were just a baby, that's to young, weren't you in Jr. High at that age, where was the parents?? Have the morale values of families deteriorated?? I'm in shock, well don't be!!" "No sympathy please whatsoever."

Listening to music is different when you're high because your ears open wider, you can hear, feel and understand the stories behind the verses. All of my senses seem to open up more on a higher sophisticated level. I can't speak for others, I can only speak for myself when I say this.

Watching TV, movies, writing poetry, songs, letters daily tasks and chores becomes Very Super Duper. My conversation becomes exquisite and intelligent to where I would use words that I never really used before.

I study, portray, visualize, become, analyze, foresee, embark upon, transform, create, reform, bestow, expose, imagine, discover, learn, teach, rationalize, indulge, must I go on people!?!

I climb to new heights, I giftedly challenge and artiscally intrigue myself on the surroundings around me an take notice of persons, places and things, and everything that I see with my physical eyes, and what I don't see with them, I can see with the growing mentality of my brain.

I love music, and I love all Genre's of music, I cannot limit myself to one category, my ears fall off the side of my head, my musical soul child evaporates if I don't hear it, play it, beat it, or feel it in some way. It is in my blood. I "Fa Real "I have to be around it.

When things finally calm down for a minute before everything started to turn funny again. I went home later that evening I didn't say a word to anyone about what I did that day. That experience was what I encountered. **"Bottom line here is that the weed seemed to helped and the pills didn't so say what you must.**

Just like my Favorite song (“I Don't Care”) that song on Foxy Brown's album Number #1 off of the Broken Silence, This album should have went triple and beyond it's means. "Foxy I Love you Girl for making that Hot Record. It was straight to the point, Cut the Chase, let me say it in big letters for all of you to read.

!! I, I, I *Don't Care!!*

1 Mo tyme for all hata'z to see

!! I, I, I *Don't Care!!*

"The Criticism Begins" Sshhhh listen, I can hear it, I hear you hypocrites in the back ground mouthin off, What does his mother think? Does she know about this? "You got your smoke on too, so don't even try to put the blame on me".

I am not, nor have I ever been addicted to weed or any other drug and/or illegal substance. I can stop at a pin drop of a dime, I can be around it and not want a puff. I don't get cravings or urges like most people in general who smoke.

I don't relapse, If I wanna smoke I'm gonna smoke truth be told. I have no reason whatsoever to lie or perform some punk copout and/or say, "Oh I relapsed", like most people do and/or say, anybody who says they quit but are relapsing for a minute, is using that as a crutch for leverage.

That to me is a straight up punk copout from a persons lips who's totally in denial, uses that sentence as crutches for their to "get-by" stigma habit which now controls them, instead of controlling their own habits themselves individually.

If you can't quit yet, don't be ashamed to say that you can't quit on your own yet, that you need help in seeking professional counseling, or time to quit or cold turkey.

There are many ways to do so, but the number 1 most important way in getting help, is that you yourself as an individual must first become responsible, recognize, approach the truth, and see the denial that is dwelling inside of you concerning the problem, habit, addiction, or whatever you wanna call it just as long as the reality of it is real. Seek God!!

Some people take time out and chew gum, wear a patch, go to rehab, or take some type of new habit in order to stop smoking. "Again, people, if I want to do something I am going to do it. If I don't want to do it, then I'm not going to do it, it's as simple as that.

I never smoked weed daily, "I can't do it"." I'm not trying to knock or stab anyone who prefers, does or likes to smoke weed everyday. In my own personal choice of opinion smoking weed was and still is boring to me.

Everyday was not in my forte', or how bougie people say "not my cup of tea". Weed would've bored me to deaf had I smoked it everyday. "I just cannot do it, No way No how". I am an off-an-on kinda guy. I do it when I feel necessary.

If any doctors or pharmacists scheduled order a weed subscription prescription as medication for me to take responsibly on a daily basis; no matter if I started right now, yesterday, tomorrow, or 6 six years ago, (which by the way still hasn't happened yet!) I would use my prescription responsible **but!**

"Somebody just said "**Aha!!. the word <u>but!!</u> just came into play, I knew it! I knew it! I knew it all along that there was a <u>but!!</u> creepin on a come up somewhere in his speech**"

(Myles insert> *"That's right folks, I did use the word but at the end of my paragraph. I was just about to tell you why I used the word <u>but</u> before I got so rudely interrupted by my excited readers, I'll explain over, ready? here it goes again.*

If any doctors and/or pharmacists decided to order a weed subscription prescription as medication for me to take responsibly on a day to day basis; no matter if I started right now, yesterday, tomorrow, or 6 years ago, I would use my prescription responsible but!, I would partially decline (some not all of) the instructional procedures that the label has legislated, informing me how, when, and/or in what way upon taking it.

Which means to me in my own odd laymen's terms for you to understand better. If the label said, "To help calm or relax Tourette's, roll and smoke 2 joints or blunts 3 times a day for a month or so until my next appointed visit for refills.

Okay you guys this is where I'd break in and say that-"that will never happen!". "I would not follow those directions if done were given to me. What did I just say to you on another page, at the very bottom in that small paragraph about smoking it everyday.

"Need I repeat myself?, I guess I do" "I do not smoke everyday because it's boring to me. Are you happy now! When and if I buy weed, Not once in my being have I ever smoked it all (a nickle or dime bag by myself, and no I didn't say that I find people to smoke with me if I am bored or need some help cause I don't. I simply give it away, throw it away, or save it for some other time. I aint stingy like some folks, nope I'm courteous.

I never really could finish a whole joint or blunt by myself. But if I feel like smoking the whole thing, just for the heck of it I will. After inhaling the first 4-5 pulleys I'm bullet, and by the time the joint or blunt gets about an 1½ to 2inches in length as soon as its lit not even near the middle, I may or may not pull it 3 more times before I put it out. It doesn't take much for me to get bullet. Weed helps me in a lot of ways many people will not ever understand.

I have told my mother about how it helps me, but like any real, loving, caring, cherishing, God Fearing, and no nonsense "I aint the one type of parent that she is, didn't agree and wasn't having any beef about it. When I did it, I did not do it around her.

I remember a funny time, that today is still so memorable every time I think about it. Back in the early summer year of 2000, we lived in a suburban area near Nashville. TN. For several years we stayed in an apartment complex, in a nice upper/middle class suburb dubbed (G.O.R) G.O.R is what everybody really liked to call it. If any one asked you where you stayed at you said "G.O.R" It is a very nice community.

It has it's very own basketball court, volleyball court, swimming pool, 2 playgrounds, green thangs. Green thangs were this big green steel generators that looked like huge green boxes, which kept all of the hidden wires for lights, cable, etc. Each individual apartment complex section had a green thang.

My brother and I used to sit and bang on them alot, all of the young and older kids would sit and bang on the green thang. There's wasn't one single day that passed by without the green thang being untouched. No matter the weather or situation, cloudy or rainy days, sleet, hail, snow, tornados, thunderstorm watches, hurricanes, earthquakes, we were on it.

Rapping, freestylin, spittin game to a girl or guy you liked, smoking weed on it, sleeping on it, playing hide-n-seek, fighting, talking out our daily problems or dislikes, drawing, eating, coming together as friends, if you had a bad day you'd have to go and chill on the green thang.

The most popular green thang that everyone loved to use was on top of the hill front of our apartment, on the far right curb across the street from the big trash dumpster next to our building where we used to live. Almost anything imaginable. I speak for everyone who's ever had a personal experience with the green thang by saying that It was personal family member to my brother, me, and everyone else who knew the Green Thang.

I bet that you guys are really buggin out and want to know about this Green Thang. Yall are probably sayin "Yo' he can't be serious can he? What's the deal with this thing that he calls the green thang? Why is he so serious and fascinated when he talks about it, he's written a page and a ½ about this green thang, and he's still rambelin on-an-on.

I want to know the history bout this green thang, How can I learn and/or gain more information about the Green Thang. Are there any books, photos, memorabilia, or documentaries that talk about or explore the very essence of it's nature. Where can I get one? How much does it cost? Is it expensive? Will I have to travel, and how far will I have to go to see it? I had to say all of that, because it meant a lot to me and to everyone that was brought up or will be brought up with the Green Thang! A lot of you are pondering what is the Green Thang, one day soon, I will make a documentary of the Green Thang!

Just go ahead and say it, just say that "I'm insane in da membrane."

Thank You Green Thang 4 Every Single Memory!! *1LUV 4ever*

Big Up Green Thang!!

One day I was outside was chillin on the green thang getting blazed with one of my triplets homies and I were smoking, my mom's was on a mission runnin some business affairs, me and my brother had spent a weekend over a friends house. We chillin on the Green Thang. Mom's comes home, I told my homie triplet that "I'll be back shortly. I go in the house, my brother comes home for a minute, he looks and laughs at me cause he knows what I was doing.

Our mother would never know when I was high, but as for my brother, He would always know, I didn't have to say anything. He kept it under wraps for me for along time until that one particular day were he says "just tell her man, tell her that you got some new medicine that helps you stop buppin. Buppin is what my brother likes to call it. She asked me was I high? I said yes and it does help way better than the pills did.

I told her to have a seat on the couch with me to, observe me as I sit comfortably and not make any sudden movements or noises for the next 10 minutes. I sat for 20 minutes and she laughed and couldn't believe that my brother and I were telling the truth about how the weed helps me as for medicine terms in the physical sense.

After the moment was over, we all laughed, my brother told mom's that he knew about it all along and didn't wanna tell her cause she'll spazz out and she did she went off!! She said how do you feel?, what does it make you feel like? and I looked at her and said" "I don't feel like any different than the way that I came in here other than it calms and relaxes my Tourette's".

Then, she said you shouldn't be smoking it", again I told her that It helps my Tourette Syndrome, I don't get any side effects other than the regular affects weed creates when you smoke it. It was totally different taking hadol, the pills that I dreaded to take so much.

I gave her and my brother some love and went right back out the front door in which I came, went outside and combed the G.O.R in search of my triplet homie. As soon as I found him, we went back to the green thang, I told him that I had some news for him, he's rollin up again, gave him the 411 as we got bullet, and enjoyed the rest of the day. end of story.

A lot of people that I have smoked with would in their own individual way express what it was like being around me when we all get high, It does help me out. Go right ahead and ask them I don't care. Somebody, somewhere saying man this guy is silly he so bold with telling you about his many run-ins with Ms. Mary Jane.

I'm just trying to be as real as I can be about myself, and share some insight with you people. You are more then welcome to your own opinion.

10

I don't know any other way of sayin this but in my own quoteabble way **I truly Thank God for granting me this moment of clarity for not walking with me, but carrying me man!!** Through all that I have been through thus far, you people just don't know how easy it was for me to score guns and drugs and hug the block. Especially for someone like me, don't let the Tourette's or nice guy mode of me cloudy up your thinking process.

Many times over I pondered the streets raising me instead of my mom's. Pretty soon, I'll be living on my on ten toes, I'm a twenty plus male living with his mother, but not for long who could've had everything by now from hustling, but I took a different route, trusted God and waited on my money!

Big up to everyone that wanted and didn't want me to hustle. Big up to any hustler maken moves, I'm wrong for saying it but **"I Don't Care"** cause this whole world has crazy things going on from babies suffering, dying, left at birth not wanted, abused grown ups, churches poppin up on every block, twisted politics, racial issues still broadcasting among people, rich getting richer, poor gets poorer, yall know what I mean.

No father for me or my brother, no family support, mom's being the only physical income, trusting, depending and leaning on God for anything and everything, not getting help from others the way help should be given and that's with realness, a warm heart, a given attitude, not looking for attention or recognition, and being straight up real not fake.

The only way to have a better life is to struggle and enjoy and understand the hard times that you've went through to get where you are now or want to get to later on in life. You have to struggle, I mean **"A Real Struggle"**, that put you through Hell on earth," not some diet struggle that you can pinch off 2 Or 3 days of so much pain from time to time and then say okay I had enough of this, I'm ready for the good life now, "Beam me up Scotty!!" It aint that easy buddy.

Anybody that was born or raised with a silver spoon in their mouth doesn't know or have even the slightest idea what hard is.

Getting your antique doll put away, or haven that $1500 allowance taken from you for that week doesn't cut it. Wearing the same draws for so many days, holes in clothes can't by this or that, can't go hear or their, seeing people who money flash cash in ya face. But people who do have it or have had it, who won't help someone else have or get it won't have it any longer cause **the first will be last and the last will be first period.**

I think I am done I don't really know what else to say. This is my first book that I have ever written, typed, produced, whatever the terminology is that's used for a first time author.

Will I make anymore books after this you say? Well, I don't know? Anyway I hoped that you have enjoyed some of my personal business for your personal means of pleasure and/or insight to help you.

"Let me make this simple for you all to understand." I have God's name referenced in my book many times simply because he has given life and carried me through a lot of ups and downs daily. I'm definitely not trying to preach to you guys, "**I just Love, Ask, Depend, Look to the Sky and Lean on Him and only Him all day-everyday and only Him for whatever it is that I need.** I am just me everyday, I've always have been and always will continue to be me.

This whole world is twisted crazy, and it will never see peace on earth. It will only be right whenever our creator decides to erase what he has created. Say what you must,

$ I Don't Care $

~Love, Peace-N-Hair Grease Yaw~

God is Very Real

Questions, Answers
&
Comments

I have a Question, Answers & Comments Section for you to express how you feel about the book and/or you can email me at: MylesW33@aol.com

Q? <u>Did you like my Book? Yes/No Tell the Truth</u>

A._____

_____

_____

_____

_____

_____

_____

_____

_____

Q? <u>What did you think about my story?</u>

A._____

_____

_____

_____

_____

_____

_____

_____

Q? <u>Would you recommend this book to anyone else that you know?</u>

A._____

_____

_____

_____

_____

_____

_____

_____

_____

Q? Will you readers Induct or honor this book as a new family member in your personal collection of readable materials?

A._____

_____

_____

_____

_____

_____

_____

_____

Q? What subjects would you have liked to see me talk about more?

A._____

_____

_____

_____

_____

_____

_____

_____

_____

Q? Was I rude or harsh, did I show no remorse different areas of subject matter?

A._____

_____

_____

_____

_____

_____

_____

_____

Special Thanks goes to God who is Awesome!!

The Alpha & Omega. The Beginning & The End. King of Kings, Lord of Lords. The Mighty God. El-Shaddi, Jehovah Jireh, The Everlasting God!!

Thank You God For Your Son Jesus Christ! For Living Dying & Living Again, shedding your Vibrant Intangible & Priceless Blood shed for all of us and His Love 4 Us! Guidance, Wisdom, Knowledge & Understanding, Ups-N-Downs, Revelations, Conformation & Information.

To my mother Gloria and my brother Robert. For you Guys Love & Support, Good & Bad. Good and Bad Times that we went through.

I thank Me, Myself and I Myles (You Go Boy) to life, traveling from place to place and our surrounding, as I was growing up no matter where I am or what I am doing and no matter how old I may get Thank You 2 so much! I Love <u>U 2</u>!!

To my grandpa and grandma and to my uncle One Luv!!!

To people with Tourette Syndrome and/or other disabilities hold your head up, keep fighting, stay strong and don't give up!!! You Can Make It!!

To the Tourette Syndrome Foundation thank you for having a foundation for people like me. Thank you for the support groups and the information all over the world!

To The People:

Don't ROB God People Pay That 10% Tithes & Offerings and Love One Another!

978-0-595-39058-8
0-595-39058-7

Printed in the United States
55762LVS00011B/321

9 780595 390588